KETO RECIPES FOR ACCELERATED WEIGHT LOSS

Top 40 Quick & Easy Keto Diet Recipes to Help You Successfully Feel Healthier and Truly Alive!

OLIVIA ROSE

KETO RECIPES FOR ACCELERATED WEIGHT LOSS
Copyright © 2016 by Olivia Rose.
All rights reserved.

TABLE OF CONTENTS

INTRODUCTION

Hi there!

First I would like to begin by thanking you for downloading this book.

In this book not only do I help you understand what the Ketogenic diet is all about but also share some recipes for the various meals you will be consuming through the day. As the Ketogenic diet consists of consuming a large amount of fats, proteins and uses a low amount of carbs, it works wonders if you have been trying your best to achieve that fabulous body you have always wished to achieve.

However, do remember, while diets work in a simple and effective manner, it is all up to you. That is, it all depends on how you maintain the balance and not just eat healthy but also tries to indulge in a little physical activity at least three to four times a week. If you do not lead a sedentary life or your work does not involve too much of physical activity, monitor the intake of calories per day. If you lead a life which is heavy in physical activity, you will need to accordingly adjust the ratio of fat to protein to carbs accordingly. As per the Keto diet, your daily diet should include a higher amount of fat, a moderate amount of protein and a low percentage of carbs. While several people claim that diets are not the best way forward to losing weight, it is only because they tried and failed. The reason for them failing is not the diet but infact it is because they don't begin the diet on the right note or are unable to maintain the balance in what they eat or drink and hence the diet they should have been on turns into a disaster for them

If you eat healthy and just eat the amount of food as

prescribed, there will be no stopping you in successfully maintaining the Keto diet. You will not only feel lighter but also happy!

Thanks again for downloading this book; I do hope you enjoy the recipes I've shared!

CHAPTER 1:
UNDERSTANDING KETOSIS
AND THE KETOGENIC DIET

What is Ketosis?

Before we begin a diet it is always best to first understand what the diet is all about. In this chapter, I will explain what Ketosis is and how following this diet could aid you in your weight loss goal.

Ketones exist in every body and are little fragments of fat which are produced by the liver when the body's food intake is low. Ketosis is the process which triggers an alarm of sorts to the body cells to burn the fat produced or the ketones in a timely manner. In other words, when your diet is less of carbs, the glycogen levels in your body fall and you enter the ketosis stage. When this happens, the ketones prevent the proteins stored in the muscles from being used and instead utilize energy from all the fat stored in your body.

Ketosis is a normal metabolic process that happens in your body and it is essential that you stick to the regime and avoid indulging in that "just one" cheat meal. If you do skip a certain part of the regime to indulge in a cheat meal, you will lose all the progress you have earned. It will also take your body a few days before ketosis begins all over again in your body. You should ensure that your cheats are zero!

In usual circumstances, the body uses glucose as the main form of energy which allows the body to function. Glucose is obtained from carbs which we consume in the form of starchy food items as well as items which contain sugar. Most of the common food items which are high in carbs are bread, pasta etc which the body then breaks down into sugar. This sugar is either used by the body or is stored in our muscles and is called glucose.

Some people follow the Ketogenic diet also popularly known as the Low Carb Diet. The aim of this diet as I had explained above is to burn fat and use the same for energy instead of relying on carbs.

What is the Ketogenic Diet?

As we learned above that ketosis is when the body uses the fat stored in the body to create energy instead of relying heavily on carbs. The Ketogenic diet or the low carb diet helps to create the metabolic state in the body which then aids in weight loss.

In the Ketogenic diet, about 75% of the diet comprises of fats and fat based food items. About 20% makes up for the protein consumption in the diet leaving about 5% of the caloric intake to be received from carbs.

A study which was published in the American Journal of clinical nutrition in 2008 observed that a group of obese persons following the Keto diet for approximately 4 weeks lost an average of 12lbs. The participants in this study also mentioned that they were able to consume fewer calories without feeling as hungry as they would normally feel due to a reduced amount of carb intake.

Since our bodies are used to converting the carbs in our body into glucose, when we limit the amount of carbs being consumed, our body enters ketosis. Our liver starts breaking down fat cells into fatty acids which is then used up as energy.

The Advantages of the Ketogenic Diet

1. The Ketogenic diet works because we reduce or limit the calories we consume on a daily basis, thereby

your body burns more energy than it receives due to the caloric deficit. One of the greatest advantages of the Ketogenic diet is its ability to help the body control hunger effectively as compared to other diets.

2. The Ketogenic diet controls the blood sugar and reduces the increase in insulin produced daily. When we consume a lot of carbs such as breads or other starchy food products, the glucose level in our blood increases. The insulin then disperses the glucose which results in those hunger pangs you feel regularly. Because the Keto diet calls for a low carb intake, our blood sugar levels are maintained and reduce the hunger pangs.

3. The Keto diet allows you to eat food which satiates your hunger and keeps you full for longer hours. If you are following the Keto diet properly, you will find that on a daily basis you will be consuming most of your calories from meals high in fat and protein. These meals not only keep your hunger at bay but will also ensure you enjoy what you eat.

The Ketogenic diet is not a fad diet and neither is it something new, infact this diet has been around for years and is gaining prominence now. When the Keto diet is implemented correctly, it is extremely effective for improving one's metabolic health.

How to Begin the Ketogenic Diet

1. **Clear your House of all the Goodies** – If you are going to give it your all, you might as well begin with this tip. Clear out your hidden stash of treats loaded with sugar or items which are heavy in carbs. The kitchen drawer, your bedside drawer, the fridge, bags or your own cupboard. We've all been there! Clear it all out. Give away the food items you have to avoid to a person in greater need of it all.

2. **Read and Re-read the Guidelines** – Don't just finish reading this book and toss it aside. Make a note of all the food items you are meant to avoid, and the ones you are allowed to eat.
3. **Set a Date you want to Begin** – Help yourself by starting this during a non-holiday season or a time when you have little to no social commitments.
4. **Tell Everybody!** – Go ahead; tell the whole world if you have to, once you do, you know there is no backing out. This way people will also know what you won't be eating in case you do get invited to a last minute get together that you absolutely have to attend.
5. **Plan Ahead**– Now, when I say plan, I mean plan your meals, plan for a day in the week where you go shopping for groceries you require. Once you have a list for groceries, stick to it!
6. **Get a Keto diet Buddy** – Get your best friend, family, sibling, and colleague from work, anybody who is willing to hold your hand and support you to also partake in this diet. Incase nobody wants to join you, there are plenty of online Keto diet forums where you can get talking to people who have accomplished good health from doing the Keto diet. That should help motivate you further.
7. **Make a List** – Of all the things you can eat and cannot eat and put it up in places you frequent a lot. Begin with your fridge first, then maybe your workspace. That will make it a lot easier for you to stay away from indulging in unhealthy binge eating sessions.
8. **Write it Down, if you have to** – Get yourself a journal, make it a habit on a daily basis to write down how you felt after having a particular food item. That way, you can also keep track of how your body has reacted to the good and the bad. This will also help you track the amount of fats, proteins and most importantly how much of carbs you have consumed in a day.

9. **It is not Just a Diet** – When you begin eliminating grains, sugar etc from your daily diet, you will not only benefit short-term, but on a long-term basis as well. Don't do this if you think it is just another trendy diet. Do it for yourself and your health.

10. **Keep it Simple** – Your food does not have to represent some luxury hotel menu. Keep your meal plans simple, recipes can be quick and easy to make.

List of High Carb Foods and Beverages

The food items listed below are what drive up your insulin levels in the body.

1. **Sugar and any other sweetened food items**. Be sure to read labels and understand the various names for sugar mentioned on the packaging.
   - Sugar syrups of all kinds such as maple syrup, treacle, golden syrup etc.
   - Muscovado Sugar, Brown Sugar, Caster Sugar, White Sugar or Sucrose
   - Cane Juice, Cane Sugar, Cane Syrup
   - Caramel
   - Coconut sugar, Corn Syrup, Corn syrup solids, Corn Sweetener
   - Agave nectar, Honey, Maltose, Maltodextrin
   - Glucose, dextrose, lactose, fruit juice concentrates

2. **Grain and Grain Products**
   Bread crumbs, Bread, muffins, bread rolls
   Pancakes, Waffles
   Cold cereals
   Pasta
   Pretzels, Chips, Pizza, Crackers
   Cookies, Tarts, Pies
   Quinoa
   Cous Cous
   Oatmeal

3. **Corn and any corn products.** Corn can be found in everything in the form of corn syrup or as a preservative, so read the label carefully before you go ahead and purchase a product.
4. **Potatoes and Sweet Potatoes**
5. **Canned Soups/Stews and Ready to Eat packaged food items**
6. **Processed Foods**
7. **Beans like lima beans, pinto beans, lentils** are high in starch
8. **High Carb Beverages**
   - Beers
   - Dessert Wines
   - Non-Diet Soda
   - Juices from Vegetables and Fruits
   - Milk, contains lactose which is also a type of sugar. However milk products such as yogurt and cheese have a lower amount of lactose as the bacteria which are used to ferment the milk eats up all the lactose during the fermentation process of the cheese.

Once your body gets used to the healthy changes and switches to a healthier way of eating, it will realize that it does not have to work as hard as before when it comes to breaking down food in the system. This means that your liver isn't under as much stress as it was previously. Since your system is no longer clogged with unhealthy processed food items or food containing a high level of sugar and its by products, within weeks of beginning the diet, you will find yourself feeling much lighter and you won't be having too many food cravings as well.

Before you begin the Keto Diet, you must ensure that you have had a pantry intervention. If you cannot get yourself to do it, ask a friend or a close family member or your spouse to help you out. If you choose the bag of cookies over a handful of nuts or sunflower seeds, or fry up a batch of chips instead of preparing your cuts of meat, then you need a pantry intervention right away! Getting killer benefits out of the Ketogenic diet will need you to show discipline and commitment in sticking to eating the right kind of food.

Make the process easier on yourself by taking an inventory of your kitchen and pantry storage areas. Look through the fruits and vegetables that you have in stock, take account of your supply of Omega-3 fatty acid along with other essential fats, and determine how much protein how have stored up in the freezer.

The Ketogenic diet plan involves a process that burns up the fats in your body instead of the carbohydrates. This is only possible, however if you keep your carbohydrate intake to a minimum. Ensure that your pantry shelves are free of complex carbohydrates in the form of rice, refined flours and breads and pastas. The Ketogenic diet is one that may take some time to show effect, but once the fat starts burning up and the excess weight is shed off, you will be amazed at how easily you can keep away the weight from piling on.

An effective Ketogenic diet should take about a month to show all of its effects, if followed correctly. Most people that begin this diet plan find themselves converted to the Ketogenic way of eating and tend to stick to this diet for long duration.

If you maintain the right balance, and eat healthy, that's just enough to keep you going strong throughout the entire diet. Let's get started!

CHAPTER 2:
BREAKFAST RECIPES

It is important that you make time to eat breakfast and definitely eat well and not gobble up or starve yourself. Here are some great recipes that are quick to make and great to help you get rid of all that extra fat.

Recipe 1: Scrambled Eggs with Onions and Nuts

Serves: 2
Nutritional Values

Calories	199
Calories from Fat	23%
Carbs	6g

Scrambled eggs are a great way to start your day. Here is a yummy recipe for your famished stomachs.

Ingredients:
- Ingredients Required:
- 3 eggs
- 1 cup sliced onions
- ½ cup tomatoes
- 1 Tbspn Olive Oil
- 1 Tbspn pine nuts
- Salt and pepper, to taste

Method:
In a frying pan, pour in the olive oil and add in the onions and cook till golden brown. Add in the tomatoes and fry for 5 minutes. Remove the mixture from flame and set it aside. In a bowl, whisk the eggs well, add salt and pepper according to your taste. Next add in the onion and tomatoes into the egg mixture. Now cook the egg mixture on low flame and stir continuously until it is scrambled well. Add in the pine nuts. Remove from heat and serve.

Recipe 2: Bacon and Eggs

Serves: 3
Nutritional Values

Calories	378
Calories from Fat	30%
Carbs	35.6g

This is a quick and easy classic breakfast dish.

Ingredients:
- 100 gms Bacon Rashers
- 8 egg whites
- Pepper and salt, to taste
- 1 onion
- 1 Tablespoon Olive oil

Method:
In a frying pan, pour in the olive oil. Cook the bacon on a medium flame. Chop the onions finely and add it in the frying pan. Keep stirring until it turns brown. When the onions and bacon are cooked, add in the egg whites and scramble it altogether. Sprinkle with pepper and salt and serve with lettuce.

Recipe 3: Banana Pancakes

Serves: 4
Nutritional Values

Calories	520
Calories from Fat	26%
Carbs	55g

These fluffy pancakes are really a great inclusion in your Keto diet.

Ingredients:
- 1 cup banana
- 1 Tablespoon Coconut oil
- 2 Tablespoons Butter
- Handful of Chopped Almonds
- 1 egg

Method:
In a bowl, mash the bananas well. Add in the butter and grated almonds and blend it well. In a frying pan, heat the coconut oil on medium heat. Place the pancake mixture in the frying pan and cook it well. Flip it over to cook the other side.

Recipe 4: The Keto Casserole

Serves: 4
Nutritional Values

Calories	560
Calories from Fat	37%
Carbs	60g

Casseroles are a great breakfast option that can be stored for a few days. This breakfast casserole recipe is something that your whole family can enjoy. This recipe includes sweet potato and although too much of it should not be consumed, it provides the amount required for your daily carb intake when you are on the Keto diet.

Ingredients:
- 1 small onion
- 1 Sweet Potato
- Pork sausage
- 1 cup spinach
- 2 Tablespoons olive oil
- 5 eggs
- ½ cup coconut milk
- Dash of nutmeg
- Salt and pepper, to taste

Method:
Preheat the oven to 400 degrees Fahrenheit. Add in the olive oil, salt and pepper and roast them in oven for 15 minutes. Cut and sauté your onions in olive oil till the onions are caramelized. Next cook the sausage on medium heat. In a separate bowl, whisk the eggs, almond milk, nutmeg, salt, and pepper. Blend it well. In a baking dish, assemble the browned sausage at the bottom followed by the caramelized onions and roasted potatoes. Top it with the spinach. Next pour in the egg and coconut mixture to cover all the ingredients. Bake at 350 degrees Fahrenheit for 20-30 minutes.

Recipe 5: Breakfast Meatloaf

Serves: 4
Nutritional Values

Calories	600
Calories from Fat	45%
Carbs	85g

Eating meat for Breakfast can keep you energized for a long time and give you all the energy that you need for your daily activities.

Ingredients:
- 12 ounces of pork sausage
- 1 pound of ground beef
- 2 cloves of garlic, minced
- 4 ounces of sliced mushrooms
- 1 zucchini, chopped
- 1 Tbspn bacon fat.
- 1 yellow onion, chopped
- 2 Tbspns of dried parsley
- 1 Tspn of garlic powder
- 2 Tbspns of dried basil
- Salt and pepper

Method:
Take a skillet and place it over medium heat. Add the bacon fat to it. Add the onions and garlic and cook until tender. Add zucchini and place the lid and cook for a few minutes. Add the mushrooms and cover and cook for a few more minutes. Cook until the vegetables have become tender. Add the basil, parsley, garlic powder, salt and pepper and remove the skillet from the heat. Stir well with a spoon and let it remain. After the vegetable mix has cooled down, transfer it to a large bowl. Add the sausage and ground beef and mix it well with your hands. Place the mixture in your crock pot and press down well so that it does not crumple. Cook on low heat for 8-10 hours. Garnish with avocado and serve.

Recipe 6: The Keto Shakshuka

Serves: 4
Nutritional Values

Calories	272
Calories from Fat	32%
Carbs	37g

Shakshuka is a very popular healthy breakfast dish which is predominantly eaten in North Africa, especially Morocco.

Ingredients:
- 3-4 Eggs, preferably Omega-3 enriched
- 3 Garlic Cloves
- 3 Tomatoes
- 2 Medium or 1 Large Onion
- 1 Green, Red or Yellow Bell Pepper
- Spicy Hot Sauce
- 1 Tbspn Clarified Butter
- 1 Cup Water
- Salt and Pepper, to taste

Method:
Finely chop the onions, garlic, tomatoes and bell pepper. Heat a pan and add the clarified butter. Once the butter is heated, add the chopped ingredients to the pan. Toss around till the onions get a transparent color. If you like spice, add paprika or a Tspn of your favorite spicy sauce along with salt and pepper. Add the water to the pan and cover it. Let it simmer for 5-10 minutes. This is the sauce for your shakshuka. Add the eggs on top of the sauce, and cover the pan till you see the egg cooked. Garnish with chopped Parsley.

Recipe 7: Spinach Sausage Stir Fry

Serves: 4
Nutritional Values

Calories	350
Calories from Fat	45%
Carbs	65.6g

This is a quick and easy recipe to make, and it is sure to be a hit with the whole family. It can be had for breakfast or for any other meal too.

Ingredients:
- 2 Medium Bell Peppers (Pick any color, red, green or yellow or use 1 of each!)
- Handful of Spinach leaves
- Chicken Sausages (You can improvise and use any of your favorite sausages)
- 1 Large Onion
- 1.5 Tspn Hot Sauce
- 1 Tbspn Clarified Butter
- Fresh Parsley
- Salt and Pepper to taste

Method:
Wash the Spinach leaves under cold water to remove any dirt remaining on it. Roughly, chop the spinach, bell peppers, onions, sausages and parsley. Heat a pan with clarified butter and add all the ingredients to it, beginning with the onions. Add salt and freshly cracked black pepper. Stir for some time. Add your favorite hot sauce to this and let it cook for some time. Once cooked, garnish with chopped parsley.

Note: You can add any of your favorite vegetables to this dish. E.g., You can even add chopped cabbage.

Recipe 8: Avocado Delight Smoothie

Serves: 2
Nutritional Values

Calories	366
Calories from Fat	30%
Carbs	45.5g

This dish is a creamy combination of avocado and banana along with added nutrition of flax seeds. This smoothie is a great pick me up and hardly takes minutes to prepare.

Ingredients:
- 1 Banana
- 1-Pitted Avocado
- 1 Tbspn Flax Seeds
- ½ Cup Almond Milk (Optional, this is only to be used if you do not like a super thick smoothie)

Method:
Add all the ingredients to the blender and blitz until you get a puree like consistency. If you feel the smoothie is too thick for you, go ahead and add coconut milk or almond milk.

Serve Cold.

CHAPTER 3:
LUNCH RECIPES

Recipe 1: Spicy Chicken Salad

Serves: 2
Nutritional Values

Calories	185
Calories from Fat	30%
Carbs	24g

This is a light salad, so if you are at work, you will not be feeling drowsy or lethargic after lunch. You can also make this salad over the weekend and keep in an airtight container. Pour the dressing over it only when you are ready to eat it. You can also chop and add the avocado only when you decide to eat this.

Ingredients:
- 1-Pitted Avocado
- 1 Mango
- 2.5 Cups Shredded Grilled Chicken
- 2 Bowls of Roughly Chopped Lettuce
- 1 Bowl of Pitted Olives (Black or Green, take your pick)
- ½ Tbspn Ghee
- Paprika
- Roasted Cumin Powder
- Salt and Pepper to taste

Method:
Take a pan and add the ghee to it. Once the ghee is heated up, add the shredded chicken to it. Add the paprika and roasted

cumin powder and stir-fry for 4-5 minutes. In a bowl or container, add the lettuce, chopped mango, avocado, olives, salt and pepper. Add the Chicken to this mix.

Mix well. Add a dressing of your choice.

Note: If you are not serving or consuming this salad as soon as it is made, avoid adding the mango, avocado and the salad dressing. You could carry the dressing in a little container if you are taking this salad to work.

Recipe 2: Walnut & Green Bean Salad

Serves: 2
Nutritional Values

Calories	80
Calories from Fat	10%
Carbs	7g

This quick and easy salad is a perfect summer meal. Light and nutritious, it makes for an excellent lunch especially on days when you are over burdened with work.

Ingredients:
- 2 – 3 Cups Green Beans (Cut each bean into half)
- 1 Red Onion
- ½ Cup Walnuts
- Salt and Pepper to taste
- 2 Tbspn Olive Oil
- 1.5 Tbspn Balsamic Vinegar

Method:
1. Chop the Green Beans into 1.5 -2 inch pieces (make it easy to eat)
2. Cut the red onion into quarters
3. In a pan lightly toast the walnuts, without any oil
4. Take a large pot of hot salted water, and throw in the green beans. Let them blanch in the pot for 5-8 minutes. The beans should still have their crunch so avoid blanching them for too long.
5. Remove the green beans and put them in cold water or a bowl of ice cubes to prevent them from cooking further.
6. Mix the salt, pepper, balsamic vinegar and olive oil in a bowl. This is your dressing for the salad.
7. Mix the green beans, onion and walnuts in a bowl. Pour the dressing over and toss the salad well.

Recipe 3: Pan-Fried Chicken with Mango Salsa

Serves: 4

Nutritional Values

Calories	150
Calories from Fat	56.3%
Carbs	16.4g

The mango salsa adds a nice sweet and tangy touch to the chicken. Makes for a delicious recipe and can be made as a family meal on weekends too.

Ingredients:
- 2 Mangoes
- 1 Bell Pepper
- 1 Medium Red Onion
- 1 Tspn Paprika
- ½ Cabbage Chopped
- ½ Cup Freshly squeezed Orange Juice
- 4 Whole Chicken Legs or Breast or Your choice of cut
- 2 Tbspn Ghee
- Salt and Pepper to taste
- Ginger-Garlic Paste
- 1 Tbspn Balsamic Vinegar

Method:
Marinate the chicken with balsamic vinegar, ginger-garlic paste, salt, pepper and paprika. Keep in the fridge for 30 minutes. Chop the mangoes, onion, cabbage and bell pepper. To this, add some salt and pepper and the orange juice. Mix well and store in fridge until you are ready to use it. Heat a pan with the ghee. Once hot, add the chicken, leaving it to cook for 4-5 minutes per side. You can baste the chicken with the marinade. Serve the chicken with the cold salsa.

Recipe 4: Nutty Salmon

Serves: 3-4
Nutritional Values

Calories	371.6
Calories from Fat	32%
Carbs	7g

If you are in the mood for something with a little crunch and a nutty texture, this dish is your best bet. Fry this in a pan with some bacon fat or clarified butter and you are in for a treat!

Ingredients:
- 5-6 Salmon Fillets; 2.5-3 inches thick
- 1.5 Cups Mixed Sesame Seeds (White and Black); You could also use Snapper or any other white fish
- Salt and Pepper
- Clarified Butter, Bacon Fat or Coconut Oil for frying

Method:
Wash the fillets and pat them dry. Sprinkle salt and freshly crushed black pepper on both sides of the fillets. In a plate spread out the sesame seeds, place one side of the salmon on the sesame seeds, do the same for the other side. Melt whatever oil/fat you are using for frying the salmon. Keep the flame on medium, since you do not want the seeds to burn and the fish to be raw. Gently place down the fish in the pan, cooking each side for 4-5 minutes. Once both sides are cooked, remove it gently and let it rest before serving.

Note: This dish pairs beautifully with a baby spinach and rocket leaves/arugula salad

Recipe 5: Chicken with Veggies

Serves: 3-4
Nutritional Values

Calories	570
Calories from Fat	18%
Carbs	78g

Here is a skillet-cooked mix of chicken and veggies with a lively taste.

Ingredients:
- 1 small chicken
- 5 onions
- 1 cup mushrooms
- 2 Teaspoons vinegar
- 1 Teaspoon olive oil
- 1 cup chicken stock
- 1 bay leaf
- 2 sprigs thyme
- 2 oz bacon
- ¼ cup butter
- 2 Tablespoons parsley
- 1 Teaspoon tomato paste

Method:
Cut the chicken into small pieces. Marinate the chicken with vinegar, thyme and bay leaf for 30 minutes. In a skillet, fry the bacon till it is well cooked. After it is cooked set it aside. In the skillet over medium heat, sauté the mushrooms in a little butter for 5 minutes. Remove from flame and set it aside. Next add in little more butter to sauté the onion till it is golden brown. Set it aside. Drain the marinated chicken pieces and keep the remaining marinade in the side. Melt all the remaining butter and throw in the chicken pieces and cook well. Add the remaining marinade, chicken stock and add in the bacon. Next add in the onions and mushrooms. To this add in the tomato paste and cook for 30 minutes.

Recipe 6: Asparagus Beef Stir-Fry

Serves: 2
Nutritional Values

Calories	350
Calories from Fat	21%
Carbs	70g

Asparagus, beef, parsley and other healthy ingredients combine to make this delicious main course.

Ingredients:
- 1 onion
- 1/2 bunch green or white asparagus
- 2 red bell peppers
- 1 garlic clove
- 4 beef pieces
- 1 Tablespoon ginger
- Parsley
- Coconut oil
- Salt and pepper to taste

Method:
Finely chop the onion, red peppers, asparagus, and ginger. Stir-fry the vegetables one by one and set aside. In a wok, add in some coconut oil to stir-fry the beef strips and cook over high heat. To this add in the garlic and onion. Next add in the asparagus and bell peppers and stir fry for another few minutes. Finally season it with the ginger, salt and pepper. Garnish it with parsley.

Recipe 7: Beef Chili

Serves: 2
Nutritional Values

Calories	401
Calories from Fat	30%
Carbs	60.8g

Ingredients:
- 1 pound beef meat
- 1 cup tomato
- 4 green chilies
- 1 onion
- 1 cup olives
- 1/2 Tablespoon garlic powder
- 1 Tablespoons chili powder
- 1/2 Tablespoon smoked paprika
- Salt and pepper, to taste

Method:
First in a wok, cook the beef pieces till it becomes brown. In another pan, add in the finely chopped tomato, onions and olives and sauté it well. Next add in the chilies and the spices. Finally place the beef pieces in the mixture and cook well.

Recipe 8: Salmon with Mushroom

Serves - 2
Nutritional Values

Calories	367
Calories from Fat	18%
Carbs	75g

Salmons coupled with creamy mushrooms make one scrumptious meal.

Ingredients:
- 4 pieces king salmon steaks
- 1 cup mushrooms
- 1 Tablespoon olive oil
- ½ cup chicken stock
- 1 Tablespoon garlic
- 3 Tablespoons butter
- ½ Tablespoon thyme leaves
- 2 Tablespoons shallots
- 1 Tablespoon lemon juice
- Salt and Pepper to taste
- Parsley leaves

Method:
Sprinkle olive oil on the salmon fillets. Season it with salt and pepper. In a heavy pan, sauté the mushrooms and keep it aside. Grill the fish till it is well cooked. In the pan add the shallots and garlic and add in the chicken stock. Keep heating till the liquid is half, add in the thyme. In another pan, reheat the mushrooms with butter. Remove the salmon from your grill and top it with the mixture. Garnish with parsley and lemons while serving.

CHAPTER 4:
DINNER RECIPES

Recipe 1: Meatballs with Mushroom Sauce

Serves - 3
Nutritional Values

Calories	550
Calories from Fat	32%
Carbs	66g

This is one of the great Keto recipes that is easy to make and delicious at the same time.

Ingredients for Meatballs:
- 1 pound veal or beef
- ½ cup mushrooms
- ½ onion
- ¼ Teaspoon dried oregano
- ¼ Teaspoon dried basil
- 1 egg
- 2 Tablespoons parsley
- 1 Teaspoon raw honey
- Salt and pepper, to taste

Ingredients for Sauce:
- 1 Tablespoon olive oil
- 1 Teaspoon thyme
- 8 ounces mushrooms
- ¼ cup red wine
- 1 cup beef broth

Method:
In a mixing bowl, add in the chopped onions, eggs, mushrooms and honey. Add in the meat. Next sprinkle the oregano, parsley, and basil and mix well. Preheat your oven to 360 Fahrenheit. Make meatballs which are around 2 inches in size. Place it on a baking sheet. Cook for 30 minutes. While your meatballs are getting ready, you can start making the sauce. For the sauce, take a skillet; add in a little olive oil and sauté the mushrooms for 5 minutes over medium heat. When the meatballs are ready, put them one by one in the sauce. Pour in the beef broth a teaspoon of thyme and allow it to simmer for a few minutes. Pour in the wine and keep stirring till all the flavors have combined.

Recipe 2: Seafood Stew

Serves - 3
Nutritional Values

Calories	130
Calories from Fat	9%
Carbs	55g

Here is a rich and creamy recipe with lots of crab, fish, prawns and less of work.

Ingredients:
- 1 Pound Mixed Seafood such as Crab meat, fish, prawns etc
- 1 cup fish stock
- ½ cup red wine
- 2 Tablespoons parsley
- 3 Tablespoons olive oil
- 15 Tablespoons tomato paste
- 4 shallots
- 1 celery stalk
- 2 bay leaves
- 2 Teaspoons thyme
- Salt and pepper, to taste

Method:
In a bowl, using a fork break the crabmeat, fish and prawns and mix it well with the parsley. In a pan, pour in some olive oil and sauté it over medium heat for 3 minutes. Pour in the wine and allow it to simmer for 5 minutes. Next on high heat, pour in the fish stock and tomato paste and keep stirring. Make sure to avoid the formation of any lumps. Add in the thyme and bay leaves. Keep stirring and allow it to simmer for 15 minutes. Season it with salt and pepper. Pour sauce over the seafood.

Recipe 3: Chicken Kebabs and Eggplant

Serves - 3
Nutritional Values

Calories	179
Calories from Fat	13%
Carbs	65g

Easy to prepare, delicious to eat with no compromise in the taste, here's a recipe you will try again and again.

Ingredients for Kebabs:

- Skewers
- 4 chicken pieces
- 1 onion
- 1 red pepper
- 1 green pepper
- Olive oil
- Salt and pepper to taste

Method:

In a skillet, pour in the olive oil and over medium heat sauté the onions, green pepper, and red pepper. Add in salt and pepper according to your taste. Dice the chicken pieces. Over medium-low heat, place the chicken pieces on the barbeque. Cook it for 10-15 minutes.

Ingredients for Eggplant:

- 1 eggplant
- 2 Tablespoons balsamic vinegar
- 3 Tablespoons olive oil
- 2 cloves garlic, minced
- Dash of fresh thyme, oregano and basil
- Salt and pepper, to taste

Method:
Slice the eggplants lengthwise in half. In a bowl add the vinegar, olive oil and combine it well. Next mince the garlic, and add thyme, basil and oregano. Brush this mixture on all sides of the eggplant. Place the eggplant over medium-high heat and barbeque it and allow it to cook for 10 minutes on both sides.

Recipe 4: Chicken Lasagna

Serves - 2
Nutritional Values

Calories	286
Calories from Fat	17%
Carbs	67.5g

Rich and classic lasagna cooked up Keto style!

Ingredients:
- 500g minced chicken
- 1 onion
- 1 tomato
- 3 garlic cloves
- 2 Tablespoons tomato paste
- Dash of sage, basil, thyme, cumin ground
- 1 Teaspoon cinnamon
- 1 medium eggplant
- 2 Tablespoons olive oil
- ½ cup zucchini
- Salt, to taste

Method:
For the sauce, you need to first sauté the garlic and onion till it is brown. Keep it aside. Next pre-heat your oven to 180 degrees Celsius. Cook the minced meat and keep stirring till they are no big lumps. When the minced meat is well cooked, add in the sautéed onion and garlic into the pan. Mix in the basil, thyme, sage, salt, and cumin according to your taste. Pour in the tomato paste and cook it for 5 minutes. To this add the diced tomatoes and simmer it for 30 minutes. Slice the eggplant and place it at the bottom of your lasagna dish. Layer it with the mince meat mixture. Add a layer of zucchini slices and any other vegetable you like. Pour another layer of minced meat mixture. Bake it in the oven for 30-40 minutes. Leave it to cool for 10 minutes before serving.

Recipe 5: Chicken on a Stick!

Serves - 2
Nutritional Values

Calories	247
Calories from Fat	13%
Carbs	56g

This is a scrumptious meat on the stick recipe you are sure to love.

Ingredients:
- 1 pound chicken breast
- 1 onion
- 2 garlic cloves
- 1 Tablespoon olive oil
- ¼ cup lemon juice
- 1 Tablespoon chili flakes
- 1 Tablespoon ground turmeric
- 1 Tablespoon ground coriander seeds
- 1 cup fresh coriander leaves

Method:
In a food processor blend the garlic cloves, onions, coriander, olive oil, lemon juice, and turmeric till it forms a smooth texture. Dice the chicken into little pieces. Marinate the chicken with the mixture and set aside in the refrigerator for a few hours. Thread the chicken to the skewers and coat it well. Pre-heat your oven to 180 degrees Celsius. Place the chicken skewers on a tray. Line it with baking paper. Bake the chicken in the oven for 30 minutes or until the chicken is cooked well.

Recipe 6: Herb Baked Salmon

Serves - 2
Nutritional Values

Calories	350
Calories from Fat	20%
Carbs	5g

They say that dinner should preferably be the lighter of the meals. This dish will not only satiate your hunger but will also ensure you have a good night's rest.

Ingredients:
- 2 pounds salmon fillets (cut into ½ pound fillets)
- 4 ounces sesame oil
- 1/2 cup light soy sauce
- 1 teaspoon minced garlic
- 1/2 teaspoon ground ginger
- 1/2 teaspoon basil
- 1 teaspoon oregano leaves
- 1/4 teaspoon thyme
- 1/2 teaspoon rosemary
- 1/4 teaspoon tarragon
- 4 ounces butter
- 1/2 cup chopped fresh mushrooms
- 1/2 cup chopped green onions

Method:
Stir together the soy sauce, sesame oil and spices and pour over the salmon. Seal it in a bag or a keep it in a box and store in the marinade for 1-4 hours. Preheat oven to 350 degrees F while lining a large baking pan with foil. Lay out fish fillets in a single layer and pour out the marinades into the pan and bake fillets for 10-15 minutes. While the salmon is baking, save time, and get the vegetables ready. Melt the

butter. Add the vegetables to it, and mix to coat vegetables. Remove the salmon from the oven, and pour the butter mixture over the salmon fillets, making sure each fillet gets covered. Bake in the oven preheated to 350 degrees F for about 10 minutes more. Serve warm.

Recipe 7: Cabbage Rolls

Serves - 2
Nutritional Values

Calories	288
Calories from Fat	24%
Carbs	50g

Easy to make cabbage rolls that you can make any time. You can even make and serve these at parties. This recipe uses chicken mince as a stuffing for the cabbage rolls, however, you can use the meat of your choice, though I prefer beef mince for this recipe.

Ingredients:
- 1 head cabbage
- 1 pound chicken
- 1 red onion
- 2 eggs
- 1 Teaspoon pepper
- 1 Teaspoon oregano
- 1 clove garlic, minced
- 6 tomatoes

Method:
Wash the cabbage and remove the leaves. Peel and make a puree of the tomatoes. In a bowl, shred the chicken, add in the oregano, pepper, finely chopped garlic, eggs, and onions and mix it all well. Fill each of the cabbage leaf with chicken mixture and roll it. Place it in a baking dish and pour the tomato puree over it. Cover it with foil. Bake it at 350 degrees Fahrenheit for 30 minutes.

Recipe 8: Crunchy Baked Chicken

Serves - 2
Nutritional Values

Calories	405
Calories from Fat	90%
Carbs	10g

Quick and easy to make, this dish works well when you are back home after a long tiring day at work. You can marinate the chicken and keep in the fridge and pop into the oven whenever you are craving for some comfort food.

Ingredients:
- 1 Cup Almond meal
- 1 Tspn Paprika
- 1 Tspn Mustard Powder
- ½ Tspn Curry Powder
- Salt and Pepper to taste
- 5-6 Chicken Drumsticks

Method:
Pre-heat your oven to 375 degrees F. Marinate the chicken with the paprika, mustard powder, curry powder, salt and pepper. Keep aside or in the fridge if using later. Put the almond meal in a plate and roll the drumsticks in the almond meal. Take a roasting pan and you can use bacon fat or ghee to grease the pan. Roast for 45 minutes to an hour.

CHAPTER 5:
KETO DESSERT RECIPES

What good is a diet if it does not allow you to eat what you absolutely love? We all love desserts, however the recipes shared below contain zero or very little amounts of sugar. Didn't I tell you, the Keto diet is awesome!

Recipe 1: Pineapple Soufflé

Serves - 2
Nutritional Values

Calories	400
Calories from Fat	15%
Carbs	45.5g

Making this light and savory soufflé is easier than you think and the best part is it satiates your sweet tooth thanks to the sweetness of pineapple.

Ingredients:
- ½ cup almond meal
- 1 cup pineapple,
- 1 cup apple
- 4 egg whites
- ½ cup almonds

Method:
Pre heat the oven to 180 degrees Celsius. Chop the pineapple and make a puree of the pineapple till it is thick and creamy in texture. Mix in the almond meal. Chop the apples and make a puree of it. Repeat the process with the apple. In another bowl, whip the egg whites until it has soft peak. Fold it into pineapple mixture. Bake it in the pre-heated oven for 30 minutes. Garnish with grated almonds.

Recipe 2: **Poached Spiced Pears**

Serves - 2
Nutritional Values

Calories	400
Calories from Fat	15%
Carbs	45.5g

These delicately spiced pears can be served with crème Fraiche instead of ice cream. Since the pears and the wine add the sweetness, you do not need to add any sugar to this recipe.

Ingredients:
- 6 Ripe Pears
- 1 Bottle Red Wine
- ½ Cup Orange Juice
- 1 Vanilla Bean
- 1 Cinnamon Stick
- 3 Tbspns Crème Fraiche (Completely your decision. This is optional)

Method:
Remove the cores from the pears but do ensure to leave the stem intact. In your slow cooker add the orange juice, wine and the cinnamon stick. Scrape the seeds from the vanilla bean and add to this mix. Cover and cook the pears on high for 3-4 hours or on slow for 7-8 hours. When serving, cut the pears in half and add some of the liquid over the pears. Serve with some crème Fraiche. Do not get rid of the poaching liquid, it will always come handy. Let the liquid cool and then you can store it in an airtight container in the refrigerator.

Recipe 3: Raisin and Walnut Cookies

Serves - 2
Nutritional Values

Calories	140
Calories from Fat	7%
Carbs	37g

This is a great recipe for some crunchy yummy cookies.

Ingredients:
- 1/3 cup raisins
- 3 Tablespoons walnuts
- ½ cup almond meal
- 1 egg
- 1 Tablespoon ground cinnamon
- Dash of nutmeg

Method:
In a bowl, add in the almond meal first. To this add in finely chopped walnuts. Beat the egg well and it to the mixture. Next add in the honey, nutmeg and cinnamon. Mix it all well. Pre-heat your oven to 180 degrees Celsius. Line the baking tray with baking paper, and pack the mixture down firmly. Bake it at same temperature for 30 minutes, or until it turns brown and is well cooked. Leave it aside to cool and cut into small squares.

Recipe 4: Banana and Apple Fritters

Serves - 2
Nutritional Values

Calories	320
Calories from Fat	13%
Carbs	60g

This is a fruity dessert that you can whip up in a few minutes.

Ingredients:
- 2 ripe bananas
- 1 apple, peeled, cored and grated
- 1/2 Teaspoon cinnamon
- 3 Tablespoons coconut oil

Method:
Mash the bananas in a bowl. Grate apples and mix in with the bananas. To this add in the cinnamon. In a skillet, over medium heat the oil. Drop the mixture on the heated pan and allow it to cook well. Flip it over to cook on the other side. Cook for 10 minutes until it is golden brown at the bottom. Add extra coconut oil if needed.

Recipe 5: Lemon Tarts

Serves - 4
Nutritional Values

Calories	140
Calories from Fat	8%
Carbs	34g

These lemony tarts are all you need to fulfill your dessert cravings.

Ingredients:
- 1/3 cup lemon juice
- 2/3 cup raspberries
- 1 cup coconut milk
- 2 Teaspoon lemon rind
- 6 eggs
- 1 cup walnuts
- 1½ cups almonds
- 1½ cup dates

Method:
In a food processor, combine the almonds, walnuts, and dates till you have a coarse texture. Line the tart pan with baking paper. Press the pastry along the bottom and the sides and refrigerate. For the filling, take a pan, add in the lemon juice, coconut milk, lemon rind and honey and simmer it on a low flame for 2 minutes. Slowly add in the beaten eggs to the mixture. Stir vigorously till it forms a nice smooth texture. Add in some more honey if needed. Leave it to cool. Remove the pastry case and pour the lemon filling slowly into the pastry case. Bake it at 180 Degrees Celsius for 30 minutes. Top it with strawberries while serving.

Recipe 6: Passion Fruit and Mango Sorbet

Serves - 2
Nutritional Values

Calories	176
Calories from Fat	5%
Carbs	40g

Indulge yourself in this cool and refreshing sorbet recipe.

Ingredients:
- 2 passion fruits
- 1 mango
- 1 egg white, beaten until stiff peaks have formed

Method:
In a bowl, beat the egg whites till you have stiff peaks. Using a blender, blend the mango and passion fruit together till you have a creamy texture. Fold the egg whites into the mango mixture. Pour it into a freezer proof container and freeze for 6 hours or until it has set. While serving cut into slices and top it with mango or passion fruit slices.

Recipe 7: Keto Chocolate Cake

Serves - 4
Nutritional Values

Calories	550
Calories from Fat	25%
Carbs	66g

Nothing says dessert like a good chocolate cake. Here is a fabulous Ketogenic diet cake recipe to try.

Ingredients Required:
- 1/3 cup coconut milk
- ½ cup dark chocolate
- 5 whole eggs
- 3 separated eggs
- ¼ cup coconut oil
- ¾ cup Almond meal
- 1 Teaspoon vanilla extract

Method:
In a bowl, add in the 3 egg white and beat it till you stiff peaks. Using the double boiler technique melt the dark chocolate. In another bowl, add in the 5 eggs, the 3 yolks and keep mixing. To this add the coconut flour little by little. Next add in the coconut oil and melted chocolate and keep stirring in one direction. Fold in the egg whites into the mixture. Add in the vanilla extract. Pre-heat your oven to 180 degrees Celsius. Grease the cake tin and line it with baking paper. Pour the mixture into the cake tin. Bake in the oven for 40 minutes at 180 degrees Celsius. Allow the cake to cool before serving.

Recipe 8: Coco-Coffee Truffles

Serves - 2
Nutritional Values

Calories	200
Calories from Fat	12%
Carbs	40g

Coffee and coconut combined makes a surprisingly great treat.

Ingredients:
- 3/4 cup shredded coconut
- 1 Teaspoon coffee
- 1/4 Teaspoon salt
- 1 Teaspoon vanilla extract
- 1/3 cup macadamia nuts (or nuts of your preference)

Method:
In a bowl, add in the shredded coconut. Add in the coffee, salt and mix it all well to combine. Next add the vanilla extract. Make sure the mixture is firm. You can refrigerate it for 5 minutes to make it firm. Place the chopped macadamia nuts in a bowl or plate. Make little balls and roll it into macadamia nuts.

CHAPTER 6:
KETO SNACK RECIPES

Recipe 1: Easy Peasy Snack Bars

Serves - 4
Nutritional Values

Calories	200
Calories from Fat	12%
Carbs	38.6g

This 3-ingredient recipe makes for a great snack. Chewy, nutty and nutritious

Ingredients:
- 1.5 Cups Assorted Nuts
- 1 Cup Pitted Dates
- 1 Cup Dried Fruits like Raisins etc

Method
Roast the nuts in the oven for 10-15 minutes. Let them cool before you proceed further. In a food processor, add all the ingredient and pulse on high for 2-3 minutes. All the ingredients should have mixed well and formed dough like shape. Take a cake tin and put wax paper or plastic wrap in it. Add the mixture and press down. Let it chill in the fridge overnight or for a couple of hours. Remove the chilled dough, and cut into squares or bars.

Note: These bars store well in the fridge for a few months.

Recipe 2: Avocado Hummus

Serves - 4
Nutritional Values

Calories	200
Calories from Fat	12%
Carbs	38.6g

Since the Keto diet does not allow chickpeas, we need to find a way to have some dip with our kale chips. This Zucchini Avocado Hummus is the best dip you will come across.

Ingredients:
- 1 Avocado
- 1 Zucchini
- 2 Garlic Cloves
- 2-3 Tbspns Lime Juice
- 1 Tspn Cumin Powder
- 4 Tspn Tahiti (Sesame seed paste)
- ½ Tspn Paprika
- 1 Tspn Olive Oil
- Salt

Method:
Peel the zucchini and chop into small pieces. Add all the ingredients except the olive oil and paprika into a blender. Blitz until all the ingredients turn into a creamy paste. Drizzle over olive oil and sprinkle some of the paprika. This dip can last for days if refrigerated.

Recipe 3: Crispy Kale

Serves - 4
Nutritional Values

Calories	93
Calories from Fat	25%
Carbs	7g

This dish makes for the best healthy finger food instead of the regular packet potato chips.

Ingredients:
- 1 Head Kale, Ribs removed
- Sesame Oil
- Sea Salt to taste

Method:
Wash the Kale properly under cold water. Cut the kale into 1-inch pieces. Lay the kale leaves onto a baking sheet and toss generously with Sesame oil and salt. Pre-heat the oven to 275 degrees F. Bake the kale leaves for 20-25 minutes, turning the leaves after every 10 minutes.

Recipe 4: Egg Muffins

Serves - 4
Nutritional Values

Calories	93
Calories from Fat	25%
Carbs	7g

Perfect when a snack craving hits you. Since eggs are a part of the recipe, you will feel satiated until your next meal. This recipe makes for a perfect on-the-go meal by itself too.

Ingredients:
- 1/2 Dozen Eggs
- 1 Cup Chopped Bacon
- 1 Cup Diced Spicy Salami or Pepperoni
- Bacon Fat
- Sea Salt
- Freshly Cracked Black Pepper

Method
In a pan, add some bacon fat and lightly fry the salami and bacon. Pre-heat your oven to 200 degrees F. Once it is pre-heated, reduce the temperature to 170 degrees F. Whisk the eggs. Grease your muffin mould/tray with remaining bacon fat. In your cupcake/muffin mould/tray, add whisked eggs, the fried bacon and salami along with salt and pepper. To make this more interesting, add a dash of hot sauce to each muffin before baking. Place in the middle shelf of your oven and bake for 20 minutes until the mixture firms up at the top.

Recipe 5: Zucchini Chips

Serves - 4
Nutritional Values

Calories	32
Calories from Fat	10%
Carbs	5g

Did you know that zucchini is composed ninety-five percent of water? One hundred grams of zucchini only have fifteen calories, but on the other hand is replete with minerals, phosphorus, potassium and calcium. It protects the cardiovascular system and all its vitamins bring amazing benefits to the skin. These chips are easy to do and are great for satiating a salty craving.

Ingredients:
- 4 zucchinis
- 2 teaspoons olive oil
- 2 teaspoons dry basil
- 1 teaspoon finely chopped rosemary
- Salt and black pepper to taste

Method:
Preheat oven to 175 °C or 350 °F

Wash and dry the zucchinis and slice them in super thin slices (make sure they are really thin to get extra crispy chips). In a bowl mix the sliced zucchinis with the oil. In another plate mix the rest of the ingredients (rosemary, basil, salt and pepper to taste). Place the zucchinis in a baking sheet (in one layer) and sprinkle with the oregano mix (only one side, don't turn them around). Bake for forty-five minutes or until they are crispy (check every ten minutes to make sure they don't burn)

Note: Let them cool for ten minutes and serve and eat immediately or the chips will lose the crispiness.

Recipe 6: Beef Kebabs

Serves - 4
Nutritional Values

Calories	220
Calories from Fat	58%
Carbs	175g

This is a quick and easy beef recipe and you will love them too!

Ingredients:
- 2 tablespoons olive oil
- 1 garlic clove
- 1 teaspoon fresh finely chopped ginger
- 1 pound grass-fed sirloin steak (cut in cubes)
- 1 medium bell pepper
- 1 onion
- ½ pound cherry tomatoes
- ½ pound mushrooms
- 10 or 15 wooden skewers
- Salt and black pepper to taste

Method:
In a bowl mix the olive oil, honey, garlic and ginger, salt and pepper to taste and place the sirloin cubes inside. Cover with foil and fridge at least for an hour, the longer the better (just don't keep it for more than one day). Put the skewers in a dish filled with cold water at least for thirty minutes before grilling or else they will completely burn. Cut all the vegetables into cubes, the same size you cut the beef (all vegetables except the cherry tomatoes that are small already). Insert the vegetables and the meat in the skewers and grill on high heat for ten minutes. Turn occasionally and let rest for some minutes before serving

Recipe 7: Shrimp Carpaccio

Serves - 4
Nutritional Values

Calories	220
Calories from Fat	58%
Carbs	175g

Shrimps are high in protein and low in calories. They are a big source of Vitamin D and are replete with Omega-3 fatty acids. They are so nutritious, and this is why they are included on the Keto Diet. This recipe is another great way to enjoy this sea deliciousness, I'm sure you will love it.

Ingredients:
- 12 big shrimps
- 1 tablespoon olive oil
- ¼ cup finely chopped onion
- 1 chopped green chili (optional)
- 1 grated carrot
- 2 tablespoons finely chopped ginger
- 1 orange
- 1 tablespoon lemon juice
- Salt and black pepper to taste

Method
Wash, peel and devein the shrimps. Fill a pot with water and bring to a boil. Make sure there's enough water to cover the shrimps completely. While the water is boiling, with a sharp knife open the shrimps in half (vertically, making a butterfly shape). Throw the shrimp into the boiling water and bring to a boil again (only for one or two minutes). When you start seeing bubbles in the water remove from heat and drain using a strainer. Put the shrimps on a paper towel so they dry completely while you do the rest of the cooking. Heat the olive oil and stir fry the onions and ginger, remove from heat

when they are ready (for about five minutes at medium heat). Squeeze the orange and mix the juice with the lemon juice, season with salt and black pepper to taste. Cut a kitchen plastic bag by half and put it over a cutting board. Place all the shrimps in one layer and cover the shrimps with the other half of the plastic bag. Using a rolling pin flatten the shrimps and then move them to a shallow dish. Put the grated carrot on the center of the dish; sprinkle the shrimps with the green chili, the onion stir fry and the lemon-orange sauce.

Recipe 8: Fruit and Nut Salad

Serves - 4
Nutritional Values

Calories	220
Calories from Fat	58%
Carbs	175g

Replace your cravings for processed sugars with this nutty and fruity salad.

Ingredients:
- ½ cup walnuts
- ½ cup pecans
- ½ cup almonds
- ½ cup dates
- ½ cup raisins
- ½ cup apple
- ½ cup banana
- 2 Teaspoons lemon juice
- 1 Teaspoon cinnamon

Method:
In a bout roughly chop up the dates. Next dice the apples and bananas. Add in the pecans, almonds, dates, raisins, and walnuts. Combine the nuts and fruits well. Add in the cinnamon and lemon juice and stir well.

CONCLUSION

Thank you again for downloading this book!

We hope this book was able to help you to understand what the Ketogenic diet is all about and also helped you in planning your meals with the recipes shared.

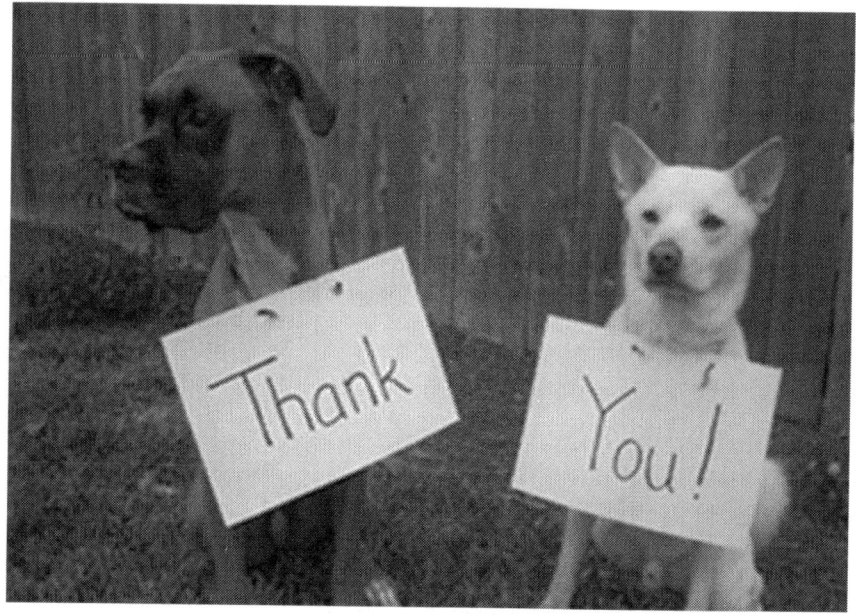

Finally, if you enjoyed this book, then I'd like to ask you for a favor, would you be kind enough to leave a review for this book on Amazon? It'd be greatly appreciated!

Click here to leave a review for this book on Amazon!

Thank you and good luck!
Olivia Rose

Made in the USA
Middletown, DE
04 June 2016